Sexual choices:
Normal sex will give you joy and kids

Abnormal and deviant sex will give you mental and physical grief.

Sexual choices will affect your whole life!
It is all explained in simple language.

HUMANS CAN LEARN A LOT FROM THE ANIMAL SEXUAL BEHAVIOR

BY S. ELIA

WHAT IS THE NATURE'S PURPOSE
OF THE NORMAL SEXUAL
ACTIVITY? PROCREATION!

HUMANS CAN LEARN A LOT FROM
THE ANIMALS SEXUAL BEHAVIOR

SEX IS FOR PROCREATION AND IT WAS
NEVER INTENDED FOR RECREATION
HOWEVER YOU CAN HAVE FUN AND
PLEASURE WHILE TRYING TO PROCREATE.

WHAT IS NORMAL SEX AND WHAT IS ABNORMAL AND DEVIANT SEX

Disclaimer:

this book is for information only. The views
expressed are those of the author alone . Should
the reader needs expert advice ON ANYTHING, he
or she should consult an expert of that field.
Ultimately The reader is responsible for his or her
actions.

Introductory statement.

These are the views of the author   . The author's
views are based on the natural laws of sexuality
that most of the animals practice in their daily
lives. In the animal kingdom , in which humans
are included , The natural law of the sexual activity
is for procreation, for making new babies, and it
was never intended for recreation.
Every one is entitle to his or her opinion and
whatever consenting adults decide to do in their
own bedrooms is their own business and nobody's
else. Whether they practice normal sex, abnormal
sex or any other kind of sexual activity ,it is their

own choice and they can do whatever they want, as long as they are consenting adults and do not use   normal or abnormal sexual activities to abuse anyone else and especially the young and vulnerable.

CONTENTS

1) prologue
2)male sex organs and the role of the male penis.
3) does the size and shape of the penis matter?

4)TESTIS function
5)FEMALE SEX ORGANS
6) OVARIES PURPOSE AND FUNCTION
7) PURPOSE OF VAGINA
8) SHAPE AND SIZE OF VAGINA
9) PURPOSE OF THE NORMAL SEXUAL ACTIVITY
10) SEX IS FOR PROCREATION AND WAS NEVER INTENDED FOR RECREATION .
11)NORMAL SEXUAL ACTIVITY IS FOR PROCREATION,
IN OTHER WORDS TO MAKE A BABY.
12) Normal sexual activity for sexual pleasure.
13) REPRODUCTION OF BABIES:
14) The chromosomes of the spermatozoa determines the sex gender of the baby during conception.
15)Planning for healthy babies
16) NORMAL SEXUAL ACTIVITY
17) SEXUAL ACTIVITY AND CONSENT
18) BEST SEXUAL POSITIONS
19) ABNORMAL SEXUAL ACTIVITY
20) PARAPHILIC SEXUAL ACTIVITIES
 21) Voyeurism : also called as the peeping

Tom syndrome

22)Exhibitionism:

23) Fetishism: Sexual **fetishism** or erotic **fetishism**

24) Frotteurism: Frotteurism is a form of sexual assault

25)Masochism

26)sadism

27) Transvestism :

28)Transsexuals and the story of the…PREGNANT MAN.

29) transgender and other sexual categories.:

30)pedophilia

31) fingering:

32)rimming

33)ANAL SEX :

34) oral sex:

35)Masturbation:

36) Wet dreams:

37)RAPE:

38) SEXUAL Fantasies:

39) Sexual obsession

40) Sexual addiction

41)PROSTITUTION, in other words PAYING

1)PROLOGUE

Humans have a lot to learn from animals regarding their sexual behavior. The animals do not need any sexual education like humans. The animals know how to behave in their daily sexual behavior. As a matter of fact the animals live their sexual habits according to the nature's laws. The animals instinctively know everything about sex. Their sexual organs are in clear view for everybody to see and they do not need to cover up or feel shy, timid or ashamed about their sexual organs and behavior. The animals are not preoccupied with their sex lives. The animals know when it is the right time to use their sexuality and use their sex

organs for the right purpose. The sexual organs
for any living organism is for procreation and it
was never intended for any other purpose.
Growing up in a farm with many kinds of animals,
I had the privilege to observe the simple life of
many animals .The animals live according to the
laws of nature. The main purpose of the animals is
to survive by eating nutritional foods and
procreating for the continuation of their kind. The
animals do not have to go to school and learn how
to read, write, how to live or how to breed. The
animals are instinctively programmed   for
everything, what to eat, what to avoid, what to
drink and when to breed when the animals are
matured and ready to reproduce. The animals have
the breeding season for the matured animals and
they never try to force any immature animal to
have sex just for pleasure. When a female animal
is mature and in heat , it produces special
hormones that the male animals can detect in the
air.
 The definition of heat period in animals is the
period in time when an animal/mammal (female) is
ready to have sex. Without being in heat period
the female will not mate with any male . Sex for the
female animals is just for procreation, period.

The animals are following the nature's laws for

sexual activity and the nature's laws is just for procreation and nothing else.
The humans do not follow the nature's laws for sexual activity, but they have sex anytime they want, just for pleasure and not necessarily for procreation and even abnormal and deviant sexual acts.

2)MALE SEX ORGANS and the role of penis

The male sex organs are the two testes which
produce the male hormone testosterone and the
spermatozoa, which in reality are the seeds for the
production of babies when the spermatozoa   meet
a suitable ovum in the female   uterus.

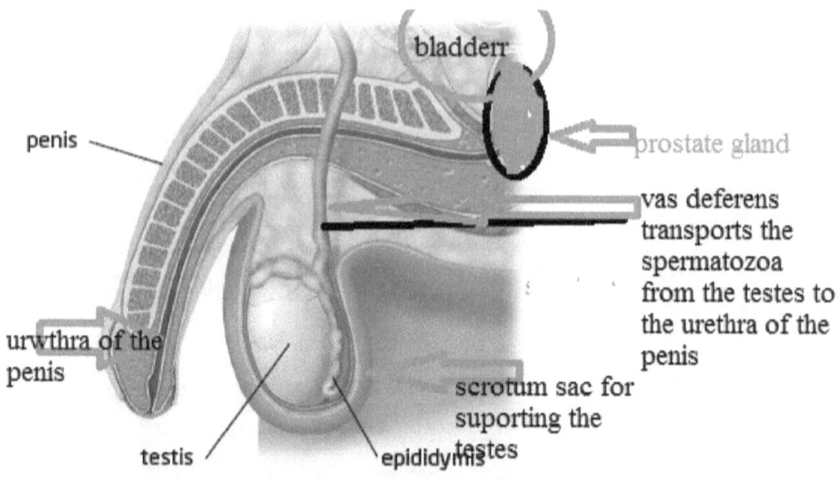

The role of the male penis.

The male penis is made in such a way to fit into the
female vagina where the sexual act takes place. The
penis role is to deliver the spermatozoa produced
in the testes through the penis urethra to

the female vagina. During the sexual activity, the
spermatozoa in their quest to find and fertilize the
female egg, leave the testes, travel through the
tube called vas deferens and through the penis'
urethra are deposited in the vagina in front of the
cervix of the female uterus. Once the spermatozoa
are placed in front of the cervix, they race through
the cervix opening , enter the uterus and seek the
female egg to fertilize it. That is the ultimate goal

of any spermatozoa. If the spermatozoa do not find any egg in the uterus , enter the fallopian tube where the egg is suppose to come out to enter the uterus. Many eggs are fertilized in the fallopian tubes and sometimes are stuck in there causing an embryo to develop there and is called an ectopic pregnancy .An ectopic pregnancy , also known as tubal pregnancy, is a pregnancy that develops outside of the uterus. This occurs when the fertilized egg from the ovary does not reach the uterus to implant itself in the uterine wall . The result of this conception in most instances do not survive. Ectopic pregnancy is treated by medical professionals by removing the fertilized egg as soon as possible before the fertilized egg grows to an embryo and causes damage to the fallopian tubes and become a medical emergency..

In conclusion, the male penis is the messenger that delivers the spermatozoa from the testes to the vagina for the main purpose to seek and fertilize the female egg for the creation of a new baby, a new life!

3) does the size and shape of the penis matter?

The size and shape of the penis varies from person to person. Penis size is unique to that

particular person that has it and not two penises
are alike. Human penises vary in size on a number
of measures, including the length, circumference,
when flaccid and

erect. There are several factors that lead to minor
variations in a particular male, such as the level of
arousal, time of day, room temperature, and
frequency of sexual activity. While some men pride
themselves for their above-average size, and others
feel insecure about the size of their penis , the truth
is that the vast majority of men have more than
enough penis bulk and length to sexually perform.
The average erect penis is a little more than 5
inches long and 1.5 inches in diameter.
 Some men have big penises 7 to 8 inches but
that   can be a disadvantage as a big penis and a
small vagina will cause damage to the woman's
genitalia. Besides the penis role in the sexual act
is to transfer the spermatozoa from the testes to the
vagina. That can easily be achieved whether the
penis is three inches or   seven inches , as long as
a strong erection can be achieved.

***If the penis is too big, more than six inches long,
it is advisable to use a foam ring around the penis
base to prevent any injuries to the female
genitalia during the sexual act.***

When it comes to the sexual activity for procreation purposes , the quality of the spermatozoa is more important than the size of the penis. No matter if the penis is small or big it can still do the job to transfer the spermatozoa to their destination.
When the sexual act is for sexual enjoyment,   it is a man's confidence, enjoyable personality, and attraction that are strong predictors for sexual satisfaction than the penis size.
In conclusion , whatever size of penis you have ,it is a valuable gift you have , be proud of what you have and never compare it with anybody's else.
You are unique , take good care of your penis and be careful where you put it.

4)TESTIS function

The testicles are the main sexual organs that are responsible for the production of the spermatozoa, in other words the seeds that will fertilize the female eggs and produce a new baby!
The **testicles** are an important part of male physiology that
 function as the main part of the reproductive system and the male   endocrine system. The testes are located in the groin region of the male body outside the body cavity ,just under the male penis. Each male has two of similar size   testes and look

like two small eggs enclosed in a loose sack called scrotum.

The main function of testicles is to produce the spermatozoa and the production of testosterone. **Testosterone** is a male sex hormone that is important for sexual and reproductive development. The **testosterone** is the most important male hormone responsible for the development and maintenance of male characteristics.

The testicles are the main male sexual organs that produce the spermatozoa and testosterone . A **man without testicles** cannot produce sperm. Sperm is produced in the **testicles** in the scrotum, if there are no **testicles**, no spermatozoa and no babies. Men without testicles are, apparently, **capable of getting penis erections and having sex but they will need testosterone to keep their secondary male characteristics, such as growing facial hair and larynx enlargement for a deep voice.**

 A man without testicles is called eunuch. It was common practice in the ottoman empire to remove the testicles of men , called castration, to serve specific social functions in the sultans' palace. The sultan wanted his many wives to give birth only to his babies and nobody's else. To be sure of that , he had all the men working in his palace castrated.

To conclude the testes are the main sexual organs

that produce the spermatozoa and the male
hormone testosterone which make the man to
have the male characteristics. The male penis is
part of the secondary sex organs, in other words,
just the instrument to deliver the spermatozoa
from the testis to the vagina .

5)FEMALE SEX ORGANS

The primary sex organs of the female reproductive
system are the two ovaries which they produce the
female germ cells the ova, in other words the
female eggs, and the female sex hormones
estrogen and progesterone.
The secondary female sex organs are a) the two
fallopian tubes, for the transfer of the ova(the
female egg) from the ovaries to the uterus,
b)The female vagina for the reception of the male
spermatozoa during the sexual act and
c)the uterus for the nutrition and development of
the fertilized egg, the developing embryo will be
attached to the uterine wall during the pregnancy,
And d) the two mammary glands ,also known as

the female breasts, for the nutrition of the new baby after birth with the nutritious milk of the mother , during lactation.

What is the role of ovaries? To produce the ova, in other words the female eggs. As we see The role of the ovaries is very important because without the ovaries no eggs are produced and no pregnancy can happen without the female eggs production in the ovaries.

The ovaries, is a pair of tiny glands in the female pelvic cavity, are the most important sexual organs of the female reproductive system. Their importance is derived from their role in **producing both the female sex hormones that control reproduction and the female ovum, also known as the female eggs,** that are fertilized to form embryos.

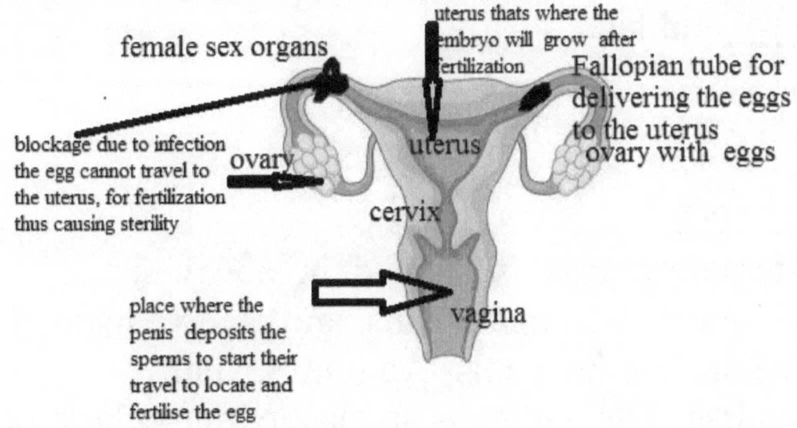

6) OVARIES PURPOSE AND FUNCTION

The main function of the ovaries in the female , is the **monthly release of eggs** to enable to conceive a baby. The ovaries also produce the two hormones, estrogen and progesterone, which prepare the lining of the uterus for pregnancy and control the menstrual cycle. When the eggs are released from the ovaries, travel through the fallopian tube to   enter the female uterus for fertilization by the male sperm and produce a baby. *So the main function of the ovaries is to produce the female eggs, and when these eggs are fertilized by the male spermatozoa a new life is created in the new fertilized egg, called initially*

embryo and later a baby.

7) PURPOSE OF VAGINA

The female vagina is shaped in a way to
accommodate the male penis and receive male
sperms during the penis - vagina sexual
intercourse. The vagina is an elastic, muscular tube.
It starts at the cervix of the uterus and ends at the
vulva, the outside opening of the vagina. It is about
6 to 7.5 centimeters (2.4 to 3.0 in) wide, and **9
centimeters (3.5 in)** long. During sexual
intercourse and childbirth, the vagina gets wider
and bigger. Because of it's structure and elasticity,
it can increase 200% and still recoil back to normal.

8) SHAPE AND SIZE OF VAGINA

Not all vaginas are the same shape or length . Like
the male penis the vaginas come in all shapes and
sizes. Usually the opening of the vagina is covered
with a thin layer of tissue called hymen when the
woman is virgin. This tissue is usually present in
childhood and early adolescence, but can be torn
away by various activities, including sexual
intercourse.

The size or length of the vagina or if it has a

Once the sperms are deposited in the vagina near the opening of the cervix, which is the opening to the uterus, the sperms race through the cervix and enter the uterus in search of the female egg to fertilize it. So in reality the vagina facilitates the reception of

sperms from the penis for fertilization and that's a very important job.

9) PURPOSE OF THE NORMAL SEXUAL ACTIVITY

The real purpose of the normal sexual activity is the fertilization of   the female egg by the

male sperm and create a new baby.
<u>The ONLY normal sexual activity is the vagina-penis sexual act. That is the only way for a female egg can be fertilized by the male spermatozoa and create a new life in a new baby!</u>

of course now a days they can have in vitro fertilization of the female by the male sperm in the lab , but that is not the natural way.

10) SEX IS FOR PROCREATION AND WAS NEVER INTENDED FOR RECREATION .

Nature with all its wisdom ,created the male penis in a way to fit perfectly in the female vagina so that the male sperms arrive safely from the testes to their intended destination during the sexual activity, for the fertilization of the female egg and the creation of a new baby. No other act with any other organs can accomplish this very important process of the fertilization of the female egg and the creation of a new life with all the necessary

support system for its survival.   The sexual activity was never
 intended for recreation or anything else. The sexual act is just for procreation, to make new babies fro the continuation of life. In the animal kingdom, which humans are members too, use the sexual activity strictly for procreation and nothing else. However humans forgot the main purpose of the sexual activity and use the sexual activity for recreation more often than for procreation. As a result of this, humans forgot the basic clues when the females are in heat and ready to conceive. There are a lot of taboos and misinformation about human sexuality. There are a lot of books written about sex, some of them from the so called sex experts, but in reality it is always the authors views , ideas , personal beliefs and even practices.

In reality only the nature's way is the real purpose of the sexual activity, something which all animals , except humans are practicing. The nature's way is the sexual activity of the male penis to female penis intercourse for procreation.
 Any other sexual activities with other parts of the body, is not the intended purpose of sex.

Normal sexual activity with the male penis and female vagina can be done for pleasure and has psychological and physical benefits but only when it is consensual by both parties and enjoy the company of each other. Sex and intimacy can

11)NORMAL SEXUAL ACTIVITY IS FOR PROCREATION,
IN OTHER WORDS TO MAKE A BABY.

In the animal kingdom all animals except man have sex only when the female is in heat and ready to procreate, and that's the nature's purpose of the sexual activity . However humans have sex for procreation and   more often for sexual pleasure .
Most humans marry and want to have kids and a family and that's
 how the human society was and still is functioning most of the time.
When people decide to have kids they should plan to have their kids and how many kids they want . The most important thing should be to find a suitable partner for having kids with. Kids is a long term commitment and once you have them you are responsible for those kids at least until they are 18 years old. But the fact is that the parents responsibility is a life long commitment. You should find a partner you like , you have the same lifestyle and with time to have a loving

supporting relationship. You respect and support each others wishes and you work towards having a happy home life. that's what kids need, to grow in a loving safe home environment.

Once you decide that you are ready to have kids, you plan your sexual activity around the ovulation time, that's when the woman produces the female egg. Without the female egg present you cannot have a baby. You always have a normal sexual intercourse, with the man's penis and the females vagina. That is the only sexual activity that has the possibility to result in pregnancy when the male spermatozoa meet and fertilize the female egg in the uterus or fallopian tube. You continue to have normal penis to vagina sexual intercourse around the woman's ovulation time until you finally achieve your desired goal, to have babies.

If the sexual organs are working properly you will be blessed with as many babies as you want . You will complete the nature's purpose of procreation.

12) Normal sexual activity for sexual pleasure.

Nature's purpose for the sexual activity is for

procreation, but humans more often are having intercourse just for sexual pleasure , and that is ok. Besides not all normal sexual activities, male penis to female vagina produce a baby.
The important think to remember that sexual intercourse is a normal activity for pleasure . It is the so called the adult games.
As long as is done with a CONSENTING partner you like and you both have pleasure, it is a normal enjoyable sexual activity . It is even considered therapeutic to have a pleasurable sexual activity with a loving partner. Any coerced, not consenting, sexual abuse or not willing participant is not a normal sexual activity , even if it is male penis to female vagina. Sexual activity with a non consenting participant is a sexual assault and it is a crime.

13) REPRODUCTION OF BABIES:

The reproduction of human and other animals' babies   is a simple process. Nature provided all the necessary requirements and support for the reproduction of babies. But in order to be able to start the process of procreation during the sexual

activity, both the male and the female have to be sexually mature. When they reach puberty, and are able to produce sperms by the male and ova (eggs) by the female they can make babies naturally with the normal intercourse. The female is sexually mature when she starts to ovulate and have monthly period(menstruation,) which can be as early as 11 years old in some girls , others a few years later. The boys sexually mature around 13-14 years old but they do not
 have any periods like the girls do ,instead, the boys start to have facial hair , strong muscles and deep masculine voice. The sexually mature boys start to produce spermatozoa in their testes and the sexually mature females start to produce eggs in their ovaries and develop breasts. A female is able to get pregnant once she starts ovulating. When a girl starts having periods it is the sign that she has started ovulating.

Another requirement for the ability to make babies is that   the sexual organs both in the male and the female are in good working order without any obstacle or obstruction. Any blockage or obstruction in any of the sexual organs tubes will prevent the desirable result to happen. Due to the fact that the female ovulates once   a month, it is important that the sexual act takes place around the time of ovulation, the release of the female egg. Otherwise if no

<u>female egg is present, no fertilization can take place and no baby!</u>

Spermatozoa are formed in the testes   and are the male 'seeds' that contribute to starting a new life. The living spermatozoa look a like tadpoles and usually are good swimmers when they   search for the female eggs after they are deposited in the female vagina by the male penis.

When a female is born she carries thousands of ova or eggs ready to use when she becomes sexually mature .Once a month, the female releases an ovum (one egg) or sometimes two (ova) .

 These eggs are the female 'seeds' that, along with sperm, create a new life.

When the spermatozoa are ejaculated from the penis in the vagina during sexual intercourse, they swim up the vagina, through the cervix into the uterus and then into the fallopian tubes of the female. These sperms are looking for an ovum (or egg) to fertilize.

If an ovum has been released, and the couple have sex, a sperm can unite with it, fertilize it and make the first cell of a new baby and create a new baby.

To conclude, when a sexually mature male that produces spermatozoa and a sexually mature female that produces ova (eggs) have a normal sexual act, penis-vagina sex, the penis delivers the sperms into the vagina during intercourse and the spermatozoa swim in the vagina, enter the uterus searching for the female egg and when they find it, fertilize it and create a new baby. that's it. The spermatozoa fertilize the female egg and the fertilized egg attaches itself on the uterine wall for its nutritional needs and in a few months a new baby will be born when it is ready to come to the world, a new life begins.

whether that baby will be a boy or a girl it depends entirely on the chromosome of the spermatozoa. If the sperm that fertilizes the female egg has an X chromosome, the baby will be a girl, if the spermatozoa that fertilized the egg has a Y chromosome it will be a boy!

14) The chromosomes of the spermatozoa determines the sex   gender of the baby during conception.

The Female eggs carry only an X chromosome and the sperm carry either an X or Y .
 An X chromosome in the spermatozoa plus the X from the female egg,   X+ X means that it will develop into a baby girl.
A Y chromosome in the spermatozoa   and the female egg chromosome X means that   Y+ X it

will develop into a baby boy.

15)Planning for healthy babies

If you want to have healthy babies you have to plan ahead and take some precautions. Again there is not 100% guarantee that your baby is going to be a healthy baby but by taking certain precautions you have a better chance that your baby will be a healthy baby.

what you do before you get pregnant or before you know you're pregnant in reality does have a huge effect on the health of your pregnancy and baby for a lifetime. It is imperative that you and your partner take the necessary health precautions so that you have good chances to have healthy babies. You have to have a healthy lifestyle and good nutritional foods for optimum health for both of you and the healthy of your planed baby.

You should stop smoking, drinking alcohol or doing any drugs or any other dangerous substances that adversely affect your health and your reproduction organs.

You should start eating nutritional foods and moderate exercising to keep your bodies in good shape. Healthy parents produce healthy babies. With the advice of your trusted health professional you should be taking some vitamin and minerals supplements.

 One of the most important B vitamins for fertility and healthy fetal development is folic acid or B-9. Folic acid is vital to both male and female for fertility. Doctors know that a low intake of folic acid is associated with an increased risk of neural tube birth defects such as spinal bifida. Research in 2012 found that proper folic acid intake may impact progesterone levels and low levels of B-9 may lead to irregular ovulation

For men, low levels of folic acid in semen are associated with poor sperm health. Men with low dietary folic acid are more likely to have a higher percentage of DNA-damaged sperm. Folate ,or as it is known folic acid supplementation (along with zinc) may also help improve the quality of the spermatozoa in the semen .

Vitamin E was discovered as a "**fertility** vitamin" and it is advisable to supplement their diet with vitamin e as well.

With a good diet, the proper supplementation with vitamins and the avoidance of dangerous health habits, like drugs, alcohols and smoking you will have a good chance to achieve your goal and have healthy babies.

16) NORMAL SEXUAL ACTIVITY

What is the normal sexual activity in humans?
 According to the laws of nature , a normal sexual activity is between a man and a woman with their   normal sexual organs, penis to vagina intercourse to produce the future generation of humans.
 Anything else is out of   the normal sexual activity , penis to vagina sexual act, it can be classified as abnormal or deviant act.
 The male penis was made in such a way to fit exactly in the female vagina and that's the only normal sexual activity for humans and the other animals of the animal kingdom. The purpose of this normal penis and vaginal sexual activity is to transfer the spermatozoa from the testis through the penis , to the ovum of the females in the female womb through the vagina,   for fertilization of the

ovum, the female egg, and the creation of a new baby. that's the only purpose of the human sexual activity , to produce babies for the continuation   of life. Nature   created the male sex organs and the female sex organs for the propagation of life in the animal kingdom. Anything else, other than the penis-vaginal sexual activity , is not considered a normal sexual activity. It might be called a recreational activity for sexual pleasure but that's not what nature had in mind when it created the male sex organs in males and the females sex organs in females.

 Any sexual activity with the male penis and the female vagina, is a normal sexual activity as long as it is done by consenting adults, no matter if it is for procreation or pleasure. Besides not all normal sexual acts produce a baby.

Many people have different opinions and ideas what is a normal sexual activity and they are entitle to their opinions and their ideas, but the nature's way is always the correct normal sexual activity and you cannot argue with laws of nature.

17) SEXUAL ACTIVITY AND CONSENT

Consent is a voluntary agreement to engage in sexual activity. Consent for any sexual activity must be freely given by both parties before any sexual activity takes place. Consent cannot be given by someone who is intoxicated, unconscious, or otherwise considered incapable of giving their consent, like the minors or people with mental disabilities. **Consent is the foundation of sexual activity and the key element that is missing in sexual violence**. Consent is truly a simple concept to understand, but first let's identify what consent isn't. You've probably heard the phrase

"no means no." This is true, but this expression is not adequate because there are many other ways to say no.
Sexual activity without consent is rape or sexual assault punishable by the criminal law in all countries.
 For many people, especially women, intimacy can lead to better sexual experiences because partners are comfortable and trusting enough to ask for what they desire and what they prefer to do.
When people have Intimate relationships usually give consent to have sexual activities. People should never give a blank check when consenting to have sex . The sexual activity is about having some fun while you doing it. So it is important to tell the other person how far are you willing to go and with what sexual activities you are comfortable with. If there is something that you are

not willing to do and you are not comfortable with it, just let your partner know before you go any further. If your partner does not respect your preferences and wishes , you can withdraw your consent before you are forced to do things you do not want to do. You should also respect your partners wishes and do only the things that you both are comfortable with and you enjoy doing it together.

Here are some red flags that indicate your partner doesn't respect your consent: They use the old cliché : if you love me you will have sex with me, or if you love me you will do this or that. You have to realize that they do not respect you and they **pressure or guilt you into doing things you may not want** to do. They make you feel like you "owe" them ,because you're dating, or they gave you a gift. They react negatively with sadness, anger , resentment or intimidation to make you do something you do not feel comfortable to do. If that is the situation , the best thing to do is just walk away from that situation.

Even if you gave consent to someone to have sexual activity with you, if they abuse you or try to force you to do something you do

not want to do, that is a sexual assault, and you should report it.

Sex is for procreation and having fun while you are trying to achieve your goals. Even if the sexual activity is just for having fun and enjoy each other, always do the things you both like. it is a two way street you both have to have fun, not for pleasing just the one party on the detriment of the other.

18) BEST SEXUAL POSITIONS

Best sexual positions are the ones that both partners enjoy and have fun during the actual sexual act. Every two people fit together differently and have their own ways to enjoy each other while they have sex. There are hundreds of ways in which male and female bodies can come together for mutual pleasure. You can do it standing, sitting or lying down. The important thing is that you both enjoy each other and have fun while you are engaging in intimating sexual activities.

For many people, especially women, intimacy can lead to better sexual experiences because partners are comfortable and trusting enough to ask for what they desire and what positions prefer while engaging in the sexual act. It is not necessary to be an acrobat and do acrobatic moves while having sex. The object is to be comfortable during the act and enjoy the company of your partner. The idea is to have fun, it is adults sexual games after all.

The most common sexual position is the missionary position .It's a simple sex position: The woman lies on her back with her legs spread and her knees bent slightly. The man lies between her

legs and guides his penis into her vagina, supporting his body weight with his arms or elbows. Both partners are comfortable with this position and if they put a pillow under the female's pelvis is even more comfortable .This position is ideal for conception purposes too.

The woman on top. The man lies face with his legs spread apart and the woman sits on top of him like she is riding a horse. She inserts his penis in her vagina and she is in control of the sexual act like riding a horse. Most women find this position satisfying and entertaining as she is in control.
You can be creative and try many other positions if you want to.
But the most important thing to remember is that

you both agree and you enjoy those positions
while you do it. Enjoyment and pleasure with a
loving partner is more important than anything
else.
Try to avoid any acrobatic or awkward positions
that can result in injuries to your body. If you are
not comfortable   during the sexual act you cannot
enjoy it. that's why you should choose the positions
more comfortable and enjoyable to both parties.

19) ABNORMAL SEXUAL ACTIVITY

Any sexual activity other than the normal male
penis - female vagina sexual act is considered an
abnormal sexual activity and it can never produce
an offspring, a baby. So, an abnormal sexual
activity is the activity that was not the nature's
way to procreate a new life for the continuation of
species. An abnormal sexual activity involves part
of the body other than the male penis and the
female- vagina for a sexual act.
*However, When the sexual activity male penis-
female vagina is for pleasure only and not for
procreation, it is still a normal sexual activity,
because both the penis and the vagina are made
specifically for the sexual act.*
Besides not all normal sexual activities , penis -to

vagina sex acts end up in procreation and a new life. The point is that nature

made the penis to fit the vagina, and the vagina to accommodate the penis for each other to facilitate the transfer the spermatozoa to the vagina, for procreation and that is why it is the only normal sexual activity .

So any other sexual activity that does not involve both the penis and the vagina in the sexual act at the same time, it is considered an abnormal sexual activity. That's the nature's rule and you cannot argue with nature.

 Anything else is called Paraphilic   sexual acts and they are defined in psychiatry and psychology, as unusual or anomalous sexual behavior. In other words abnormal sexual activity. Anything outside the normal sexual activity, penis-vagina intercourse, is called an abnormal or deviant sexual act. Period.

There are many abnormal sexual activities for the purpose of recreational sexual pleasure and they are called Paraphilic sexual activities. These Paraphilic sexual activities are defined as unusual or anomalous   behavior. The term paraphilia is often used in a derogatory way, and it's sometimes used interchangeably with sexual perversion.

However in a free society , people have full control of their bodies and mind and they can do whatever they wish as long as   it is not against the laws or harming any one else . Whatever consenting adults are doing in their own bedrooms , it is their own affair and nobody's else. It might be abnormal and harming their   health but it is their own choice and when their health pays the price they have no one else to blame. The key here is consenting adults. _**These Paraphilic sexual acts and even the normal sexual acts should never, ever, be used, to use or sexually abuse anybody, and especially the young and the vulnerable, because it is called sexual   exploitation and sexual abuse, punishable by the criminal laws of many countries.**_

20) PARAPHILIC SEXUAL ACTIVITIES

Here we are going to describe most of these (abnormal) Paraphilic sexual activities. In other words the abnormal sexual acts and fantasies and whatever people decide to do, it is their choice and responsible for the consequences .

21) Voyeurism : also called as the peeping
Tom syndrome , because they remain hidden from
view as they watch others' private parts or acts
:Voyeurism is a mental disorder in which a person
receives sexual gratification by spying on people as
they undress or engage in sexual acts or other
private activities. It is obviously that it is an
abnormal sexual activity as it has nothing to do
with the natural sexual activity of penis- vagina
intercourse for the production of babies. It is a
waste of precious time that it could be used for
something else, like reading a good book, or
learning something useful. This is a mental
fixation, an addiction to sexual fantasies. People
suffering from this abnormal sexual addiction
should seek professional help for their predicament
before they end up charged by the authorities.

22)Exhibitionism: a perversion in which
sexual gratification is obtained from the indecent
exposure of one's genitals to a stranger or a group
of people.
 Exhibitionism, also known as flashing, is the act of
exposing the genitals to another unsuspecting
person. Exhibitionism is a mental disorder and is
also a paraphilia, which is a group of mental

disorders, marked by obsession with unusual sexual practices. This

is clearly an abnormal behavior and it is called indecent exposure punishable by law. Again this is a mental disorder and an addiction to some indecent sexual behavior which is definitely weird and abnormal . People suffering from this abnormal behavior, should ask themselves what possible can they gain from exposing their genitals to unsuspecting strangers, other than   get charged for indecent exposure? They should seek professional help for their sick predicament before they end up in jail.

23) Fetishism: Sexual **fetishism** or erotic **fetishism** is a sexual fixation on a nonliving object or a body part. The object of interest is called the **fetish** ; the person who has a **fetish** for that object is a **fetishist**. In Psychiatry is the compulsive use of some object, or part of the body, as a stimulus in the course of attaining sexual gratification, as a shoe, a lock of hair, underwear , socks, etc. This is definitely an abnormal and deviant addiction. The people suffering from this deviant behavior should seek professional psychological help.

24) Frotteurism: Frotteurism is a form of

sexual assault that involves a person stimulating himself or herself by rubbing against another person who is not a willing participant in a sexual act. This is typically done in a crowded area such as a concert or on a crowded subway, bus, or train. This is an abnormal and illegal act against innocent people. It is a form of an attempted rape in a crowded place. The victims of such an assault should call out for help and report the perpetrator right away to the authorities for sexual assault. That is the only way to stop these anomalous characters from assaulting innocent people.

People suffering from this deviant and criminal behavior should seek professional psychiatric treatments before they end up in jail where they belong.

25)Masochism: masochism is The

achievement of sexual arousal or gratification by the experience of physical or mental pain or humiliation. Masochism is said to derive from a partly repressed sense of guilt which inhibits orgasm but which can be relieved by punishment so that orgasm becomes possible.

This is clearly an abnormal psychological and mental affliction and people suffering from it need psychological support for their predicament. It must be another and better way to treat their problem than physical pain and humiliation. These people are exploited and manipulated by other perverts for their own sexual gratification. Masochistic persons were probably   sexually, mentally and physically abused as children and trained to think that's what they deserve, punishment and humiliation, and that's exactly what they are looking for. That does not make it right, for any human being to be humiliated and abused, but at least it is their choice. With a lot of psychological support they might be able to get over this abnormal and dangerous   affliction.

26)sadism: Sadism is the opposite of masochism and it means to experience pleasure and gratification , from inflicting pain on others. Although there have been references to sadism as a sexual practice in literature for centuries, it was not until the 19th century that sadism was described as an actual medical condition; these days, sadism is listed as a paraphilia .

Sadism is an abnormal behavior, sexual or

otherwise. These people are sick and they need psychiatric therapy to overcome

their predicament.
Again this is an abnormal sexual activity which has nothing to do with the normal sexual activity as nature was intended it to be. Deriving pleasure and gratification from inflicting pain to others , it shows a mentally unstable and sick mind and only with prolong psychotherapy they might understand their sick intention.

27) Transvestism : Transvestism is a form of fetishism (the clothing is the fetish), which is a type of paraphilia. In transvestism (cross-dressing), men prefer to wear women's clothing, and women prefer to wear men's clothing. However, they do not wish to change their sex, as transsexuals do.
 The definition of Transvestism is the practice, especially of men, of wearing clothing usually associated with the opposite sex for sexual and psychological gratification .Transvestism as a symptom in Psychiatry can be presented as a sign of lower intelligence.
Again this is an abnormal sexual behavior like the fetishism and has nothing to do with the normal sexual activity. These people, as long as they do not bother anybody else with their abnormal

behavior , they should be left alone. It is unlikely that they would seek psychological support or treatment for their abnormal behavior.

28)Transsexuals : **transsexuals** is a person who emotionally and psychologically feels that they belong to the opposite sex.
A **transsexual** is a person who is genuinely and totally convinced their gender should be the opposite to their physical body. The modern official medical diagnosis of transsexuals is the medical term ***gender identity disorder***.
The cause of transsexualism is not known, but exposure to

hormones during pregnancy (in the womb), genetics, and upbringing may have an influence on their beliefs , feelings
and obsessions.
I was watching on television the story of a transsexual . He was born as a boy with normal sexual organs like any other boy. when he was about three years old he wanted to play with dolls and he liked to dress as a girl. His parents enabled his wishes in every way and some more. When he started school they demanded that their boy should

be allowed to dress as a girl and use the girl's
washroom because as they put it , their child had
the right to use the girl's washroom because he
was feeling that he was a girl while he had all his
male sexual organs intact. Now, nobody raised the
most proper question , that yes , the little boy had
the right to dress and feel like a girl but still he was
a boy with a penis, and by using the girls
washrooms he was violating all the other's little
girls the rights and their privacy.
Eventually the school had a special washroom for
the little transsexual to use. Eventually the boy
grew up and went for surgery to change his
manhood into womanhood and that is ok for any
reasonable person. If he felt like a woman and
wanted to be a woman that is ok for the rest of
society. It is his life and he can live it anyway he
wants.
The point here is that many boys like to play with
dolls, or dress like girls and vice versa, but it is up
to the parents to guide their kids in the right
direction. The parents should explain to the kids
that no matter what they like to dress or what toys
they play with, that's not what makes a girl, a girl,
or a boy a boy. It is not the clothes or the toys that
defines a boy or a girl. Many girls are wondering
why the boys have a penis and they don't ,but you
do not try to give them a penis. when you explain
it to them that nature decides who is going to be a

boy or a girl, and both have special roles necessary for the continuation of life , they will understand.

The boy has a penis and the ability to produce the seeds that will fertilize the woman's eggs and create a new life ,something which is unique to males and should be proud of their gender.
The girls are special with the unique gift to produce the eggs that when fertilized by the male spermatozoa will get pregnant, create a new life, a new baby that no   man can do.
In short , the parents should teach their kids from an early age to be proud of their sexual identity that both boys and girls are equally important for the continuation of life.
So , the upbringing is the most important   in the developing of a healthy gender identity.
The transsexual   individuals are born as males or females with the proper sexual organs, that's what nature provided them with . Now if they are unhappy and they want to change their gender, that it is their choice, but at what cost to themselves and society, and I do not mean monetary cost. The society lost one of its members that could procreate, have kids for the continuation of life. The transsexual lost his or her natural identity and created an imaginary world for their future, and above all they lost their natural ability to

procreate, the best natural gift of all.

Whether they still have their original sex organs or the ones they surgically acquired the normal sexual activity is still the nature's way, vagina to penis sexual act. Any other sexual act is still an abnormal sexual act with all the health dangers that come with any abnormal sexual act .   As long as they are consenting adults ,whatever they decide to do is up to them. Nobody else will tell them what sexual activities they will do or not do in the privacy of their homes.
As long as they are happy with their lives, no matter if they change their gender or not , it should be ok by the rest of the society.

A foot note that might be interested to some, is this. When you decide to change your sexual organs, there is no turning back, so it might be wise to choose what you want to change just in case you have second thoughts later… and here is why.

THE STORY OF THE PREGNANT MAN

Years ago when   Oprah still had a show, she was advertising that on a specific day she was going to interview on her live show a " PREGNANT MAN". I was very curious how that unnatural process took place, so on that specific day I watched her live show.

The man came to the show with a beard on his face and a really big pregnant belly with his wife on his side. During the show we learned that the pregnant man was really a woman(transsexual) that had surgery to get a penis but did not remove his female sexual organs, VAGINA, UTERUS AND OVARIES.

Since he(she) had his (her)sexual organs she was able to ovulate and her egg was fertilized by a male sperm and that's how he (she) got pregnant, like any other female that gets pregnant , NOT LIKE A MAN.

His story is on the you tube and you can watch it if you want.

He eventually had three kids and got divorced from his wife.

That is why I said above, "When you decide to change your sexual organs, there is no turning back, so it might be wise to choose what you want to change just in case you have second thoughts later…………" but again it is your choice and your decision and you do what you want to do.

That pregnant man, or in reality the transsexual woman, changed her mind and because she did not remove her sexual organs she was able to have three kids later on.

A footnote here is that the Tran sexuality is an abnormal mental disorder where she or he have thoughts and believe that they belong to the opposite sex and that they are trapped in the wrong body. Nature determines if someone is a man with a penis and testicles or a female with ovaries, uterus and vagina. So no matter what one thinks if they have a penis and testicles he is a man. If she has ovaries, uterus and vagina she is a woman . Nature decided that and no thoughts can change that. However if they want to change from a man to a woman and vice versa it is their prerogative and with the today's medical advances they can partially achieve that. I say partially, because even if they medically change their sex and take huge amounts of hormones to change their sexual characteristics they can never achieve to be completely what they want. No female changing to male will ever be able to produce spermatozoa and father children and no male changing to female will ever be able to be pregnant and have babies,. They can only change their external appearance,. It is their choice and they can do whatever they want and society has no say with their decision . It is their bodies and their decision and they can do as they please.

29) transgender and other sexual categories.:

There so many names for different types of sexual preferences and   abnormalities that it is very confusing even to understand what it is, even for the people that think that they belong to that group. Here is one that   describes transgender :people whose gender identity differs from the sex they were assigned at birth. Gender identity is a person's internal, personal sense of **being** a man or a woman (or boy or girl.) For some people, their gender identity does not fit neatly into those two choices. Searching the internet to find what exactly is a transgender , there is no clear definition of a transgender person, just that they have personal thoughts that they should be on the opposite sex than they are. If they are men with male sexual organs they think that

they should be females with female sexual organs. If they are women with female sex organs they think that they should be men with sexual organs of a man. When they decide to have surgery and change their sex organs, they are called transsexuals.
Just by having thoughts or wishes to be the opposite sex of what you have should not make

you anything else than what you are, just my opinion…..

One transgender woman had the perfect answer of what a transgender person is. A true transgender person has abnormal sexual organs that do not identified with a male or female's sex organs. They may have a penis , and an uterus and ovaries, or they may have testicles and no penis and vagina and any variations in the abnormality of their sexual organs.

Just my opinion , without being an expert sexologist, sexual therapist or any other sexual profession is that the description of the transgender woman above is the correct one. The other descriptions by anybody else is confusing and incomplete.

Look at the description below that is available in the internet by various authors as the definition of transgender.

"Transgender

Transgender people have a gender identity or gender expression that differs from their sex assigned at birth. Some transgender people who desire medical assistance to transition from one sex to another identify as transsexual."

Having thoughts or expressions is not enough to name a person that is anything else that what they really are.

Sex is biologically defined. You are either a

<u>**boy or a girl, a man or woman when you have normal sexual organs of that sex..**</u>

Sex is determined by virtue of one's physical sexual anatomy. It is determined by your hormonal characteristics,

chromosomes, and sexual organs.

Sexual thoughts or expressions do not define if a person is a man or a woman. But what sexual organs they have defines a man or a woman.

 When I was living in a farm , I had the privilege to observe the animals normal sexual behavior and sometimes the abnormal outcome of some animals born with abnormal sexual organs. Some animals were born with abnormal sexual organs and those animals were called by the farmers transgender animals, because they were born before their sexual organs were fully transform to either male sex or female sex organs. Those animals were not able to perform sexual acts and were not able to conceive…

So the transgender woman's description I mentioned above is more accurate than any other definition available in the internet or offered by any sexual professional. A transgender person is born with missing or abnormal sexual organs. If they decide to have surgery to remove or acquire sexual organs and become a male or female, then they are called transsexuals, like any other person that decides to change their sex organs.

 People have options and preferences these days and if they decide to do what they feel they should do, it is their choice and they can do whatever they want and it is nobody's else business. Gender transitioning is the process by which a person transitions from their assigned gender at birth and into the gender presentation that aligns with their gender identity .

 Anyway, no matter what the sexual preference or name attached to it,   a normal sexual activity is still the male penis to female vagina sexual act, whether it is their biological or the acquired by surgery sexual organs..

30)pedophilia   : Pedophilia is a psychiatric abnormal sexual disorder in which an adult or older adolescent experiences a primary or exclusive sexual attraction to prepubescent children. Pedophilia is an obsession with children as sex objects. Overt acts, including taking sexual explicit photographs, molesting children, and exposing one's genitalia to children are all crimes. Pedophilia is an ongoing sexual attraction to prepubertal children. It is considered a paraphilia, a condition in which a person's sexual arousal and gratification depend on fantasizing about and engaging in sexual behavior that is atypical and extreme. Pedophilia is defined as recurrent and intense sexually arousing fantasies, sexual urges, or behaviors involving sexual activity with a prepubescent child or children generally age 13 years old or younger

An estimated 20 percent of American children have been sexually molested, making pedophilia a common paraphilia. Offenders are usually family friends or relatives or others taking care of children. Types of activities vary and may include just looking at a child or undressing and touching a child. However, acts often involve oral sex or touching of genitals of the child or the offender. Studies suggest that children who feel uncared for or lonely may be at higher risk for sexual abuse. Pedophilia is an abnormal sexual   abuse of innocent children. It is a criminal offence in many countries punishable by the criminal laws .

Children sexual abuse is on the rise and with advent of the internet pedophilia is out of control. Governments need to take drastic measures to stop the abuse of children.

As for the abused children they have to be told that it is not their fault and that they were the victims of deviant sexual predators .

They should also be told never to be ashamed of what happened to them, and when they are adults and in control of their lives to report their abuse to the authorities and even take legal actions against their abusers . The objective of their reporting is to NAME

THE ABUSER, SHAME THE ABUSER , STOP THE ABUSER from victimizing other children, and punish the abuser for his past sexual abuse of children. The " ME TOO MOVEMENT" is a good start to send a message to all those that abuse children that they will pay for their abnormal deviant actions, sooner or later.

31) fingering: **Fingering** is a sexual act where **someone** touches another's genitals or anus using their fingers. Again this is not a normal sexual activity. They can use their finger as long as they want but it can never result in procreation. Besides the fingers can be dirty and can transfer germs causing infections. if they finger the anus and then the vagina or mouth they will definitely transfer fecal germs from the anus to vagina or mouth and cause infections.
It is an abnormal and unusual sexual act but if it

is done between consenting adults, it is their choice
and they can do whatever they want.
Again the people are free to do whatever they want
as long as they are consenting adults. If it not
consensual , then it is a sexual assault and should
be reported to the police.

32)rimming: in simple words is the use of the
mouth on someone's else anus. It is an abnormal
sexual activity that involves licking, penetrating
with the tongue, sucking, kissing, or otherwise
orally stimulating your partner's anus. It is also
called as anal-oral sex, rim job or tossing the
salad.
Knowing what comes out of the anus, this is an
extremely highly risky sexual activity. The health
authorities warn the people about the dangers of
fecal contamination of the food and water. Many
people suffered life threatening diseases by eating
or drinking food or water contaminated by fecal
materials. And then you hear that some people
use their mouth where the feces coming out, the
 anus.
Is it just ignorance of what comes out of the anus
and the dangers of fecal contamination , or people
just ignore the dangers of such an abnormal highly
risky sexual activity for a fleeting pleasure?
Anyway this is an abnormal highly risky sexual

activity and If people willingly want to take chances with abnormal sexual activities , at least they have nobody else to blame when their health suffer the consequences. On the other hand, If they are unwillingly victims of such an abnormal activity, it is a sexual assault and they should report it to the authorities. It is also advisable to see their doctor for proper diagnosis and treatment of any infection that comes from fecal contamination from this abnormal act !

33)ANAL SEX :

Anal sex is a dangerous abnormal sexual activity.

The anus is not part of the sexual organs and it was never indented for any sexual activity.

The anus is part of the long alimentary canal which starts from the mouth and ends at the anus. The purpose of the anus is for controlling and expelling the feces, the end waste byproduct of digestion. For this reason nature has provided the anus with strong circular muscles, the so called sphincters, to control the expulsion of the feces and avoid any accidental discharge. That is the real purpose of the anus and was never intended for anything else, and certainly never for sex. When the anus is used for sexual activity gradually the anal sphincter loose their function and gradually is unable to function properly and cannot control the feces causing fecal incontinence. In other words the anus cannot control the expulsion of the feces and accidents happen . People with that unfortunate predicament they have to use pampers. And
that's not the only side effect when abusing the

anus for sexual activity.

Anal sex or anal intercourse is generally the insertion and thrusting of the erect penis into a person's anus, or anus and rectum, for sexual pleasure. Other forms of anal sex include fingering, the use of sex toys for anal penetration, and oral sex performed on the anus. Any sexual act involving the anus, with the penis, sex toys, fingering , or mouth is an abnormal sexual act. Anal sex is not only an abnormal sexual activity but it is a sexual abuse of a non sexual vital organ with severe consequences. The anus was never intended for any sexual activity, therefore it lacks the natural lubrication the vagina has. Any penetration of the anus

can tear the tissue inside the anus, allowing bacteria and viruses that are present to enter the bloodstream and cause severe infections.
 The anus is full of bacteria from the feces that is expelled by the anus.
The wall of the anus and rectum can be injured or even perforated   which can be life threatening if left untreated. It is extremely dangerous to insert any sex toys in the anus which can cause severe damage to the anus and rectum ,even life threatening conditions.

Studies have suggested that anal exposure to HIV poses 30 times more risk for the receptive partner than vaginal exposure.

Exposure to the human papillomavirus (HPV) may also lead to the development of anal warts and anal cancer. **Other infections include anal herpes, anal warts, anal abscesses, anal fissures, parasites and a lot more infections depending of what bacteria and viruses are available in the fecal matter that passes through the anus.**

Anal sex is an abnormal and highly risky sexual activity no matter who is doing it.

Many people practicing anal sex end up using pads and pampers for protection from any accidental fecal discharge.

Anal sex is the riskiest form of any sexual activity and one can wonder why take such health risks for   merely some dubious momentary pleasure.

Anal sex can cause urinary tract infections and even sterility to both men and women .

Women that want to have kids some day, they should avoid this abnormal sexual activity , especially having anal sex and then vaginal sex, thus transferring the fecal germs from the anal canal to vagina. Fecal germs can cause infections to the female genitalia damaging the fallopian tubes and blocking the ova from the ovaries to reach the uterus for fertilization, thus making the ova fertilization impossible.

**People should be educated about the huge
dangers of anal sex, and if they still want to take
the health risks, at least they were warned about
the health dangers.**
If everyone start practicing anal sex for pleasure
who is going to

make the babies of the future generations. Anal sex
produces no babies, and can cause sterility to men
and women and other diseases making them
unable to produce babies and that will affect the
future of the human race .
Anal sex is a highly risky sexual activity no matter
who does it, even if he or she is the most powerful
man or woman on earth.

***Many doctors and institutions that deal with the
health issues arising from any anal sexual
activity, raise the alarm about the impending
health risks of such sexual activity.***

It is all over the internet , and all you have to do is
to search the internet about the health risks of anal
sex.

People should use common sense and precaution
before they embark in highly risky abnormal
sexual activities.

34) oral sex:

<u>The oral cavity commonly known as the mouth of the human face, has many useful uses but it was never intended to be used for any sexual activity.</u>

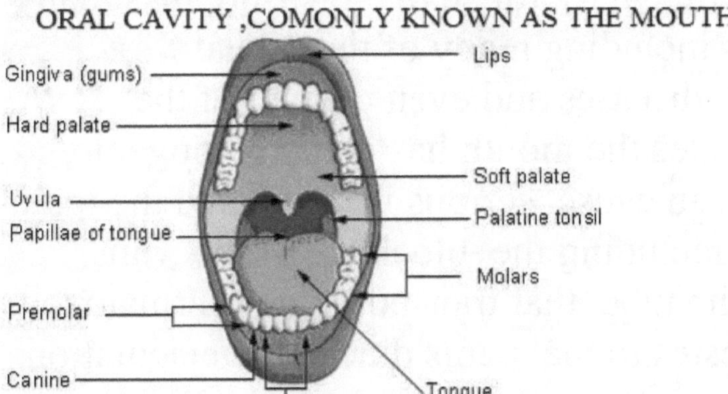

THE MOUTH HAS MANY USEFUL USES BUT NONE OF THEM WAS EVER INTENTED FOR SEXUAL ACTIVITY!!!

Unfortunately the humans try to sexualize everything for their personal pleasure.
Historically and anthropologically, oral sex is nothing new. However, social acceptance of fellatio ,oral sex performed on a penis, and cunnilingus ,oral stimulation of a vagina, and analingus ,use of the mouth and tongue to stimulate the anus, has evolved during the sexual revolution.
Before the sexual revolution, Anal and **oral sex** were considered sins because they could only be practiced for pleasure, not procreation, which is the only purpose of **sex**.
Oral sex is an abnormal sexual activity, as the mouth was never intended for any sexual activity.

Using the oral cavity for sexual pleasure has many health risks including many of the sexual transmitted diseases and even cancer of the mouth. Besides the mouth has many pathogenic germs that can cause serious infections to the male sex organs including the blockage of the vans deferens , the tube that transports the spermatozoa from the testes to the penis during the ejaculation. If both vans deferens tubes are blocked, the sperms cannot be delivered to the vagina during ejaculation and the man becomes sterile, unable to father kids.

During oral sex a lot of sexual transmitted diseases can cause serious infections to the oral cavity , including oral cancer. Then again, people are free to practice whatever they want by consenting adults and they can pay the price for their choice.

People should use common sense and precaution before they embark in highly risky sexual activities.

35)Masturbation: masturbation by men and women is widely done in the privacy of their homes. In general, the medical community considers masturbation to be a natural and harmless expression of sexuality for both men and women. It does not cause any physical injury or harm to the body, and can be performed in moderation throughout a person's lifetime as a part of normal sexual behavior. It used to be regarded as a perversion and a cause of mental disorders, however clinicians have long recognized masturbation as a normal **sexual** activity throughout life. It is considered **abnormal** only when is done in public.

Although the medical community and society in general consider masturbation as a normal sexual activity, but the fact is masturbation cannot fulfill the natures' purpose of sex which is to produce babies. Therefore masturbation is an abnormal sexual act.

With masturbation people try to please themselves in the absence

of a willing sexual partner. Again people are using masturbation for pleasure and recreational pleasure and has nothing to do with the normal sexual act ,penis to VAGINA sexual act, to produce babies and the continuation of life.

Masturbation can also be used in the collection of spermatozoa for the purpose of in vitro insemination which is another way of producing babies.

Masturbation is not as bad as some other forms of

abnormal sexual activity and in the absence of a willing partner for normal sex , it should be considered as a normal way to relieve oneself sexually, but not necessarily as a normal sexual activity.

36) Wet dreams:

During the teenage years, both males and females have   sexual dreams during their sleep, and the boys ejaculate and the girls have an orgasm, especially when they are sleeping face up.
Wet dreams occur **when you ejaculate during your sleep**. The medical term for a wet dream is **"nocturnal emission."** Most wet dreams are reported in teenage boys and young men, but it can happen at any age especially when they do not have sexual activities yet.
A nocturnal emission, also known as a wet dream or sex dream or sleep orgasm, is a spontaneous orgasm during sleep that includes ejaculation for a male, or vaginal wetness or an orgasm for a female. Nocturnal emissions are common during adolescence and early young adult years, but they may happen any time after puberty.
Wet dreams is a normal natural phenomenon, that happen to most adolescent boys and girls, and it is nothing to worry about. When they have

normal sexual activities on a regular basis , the
wet dreams will stop happening.

37)RAPE:
RAPE: Rape is a sexual assault usually involving
sexual
intercourse or other forms of sexual penetration
carried out against a person without that person's
consent. The act may be carried out by physical
force, coercion, abuse of authority, or against a
person who is incapable of giving valid consent,
such as one who is unconscious, incapacitated, or
has an intellectual disability or is below the legal
age of consent.
The definition of rape is an , unlawful FORCED
sexual intercourse or any other sexual penetration
of the vagina, anus, or mouth of another person,
with or without force, by a sex organ, other body
part, or foreign object, without the consent of the
victim.
Rape is a heinous act performed when one party
wishes to exact complete power and control over
another by having sex without consent of the other
party.
 With rape, although the sexual act might be penis
to vagina and result in pregnancy, it should never
be considered as a normal sexual activity. In order

to be considered as a normal sexual activity it should be done willingly by both parties. Rape is done

by forced for the unlawful pleasure of the perpetrator   which is the violation of the personal space and safety of the victim.
Rape is an abnormal sexual criminal act and it should be reported right away to the authorities for the arrest and punishment of the perpetrator.

38) SEXUAL Fantasies:

Sexual fantasies are just thoughts about sexual activities. Almost everyone has some sort of fantasies about sex and other activities.
However , fantasies are very different from reality. Thinking about something (or reporting having thought about it) is entirely different from actually doing it. As long as they do not act on their fantasies no harm is done. Acting on sexual fantasies can be dangerous and risky especially those fantasies about abnormal and deviant sexual activities. Such as bondage and discipline, dominance and submission, sadism and masochism. One can never predict the outcome of

such fantasies when   acting upon them.
Even if some one has such fantasies it is better not
to act upon those fantasies but just leave them as
unfulfilled fantasies.

A study appearing in the *Journal of Criminal
Justice and Behavior* found that more than 60% of
college students fantasized about sadism and
bondage and other forms of illicit sexual acts.
As long as fantasies remain fantasies no harm is
done!
Fantasies can be normal or abnormal but as long
that they remain unfulfilled fantasies no harm is
done to anybody.

39) Sexual obsession
With **sexual obsessions** people have **sexual**
thoughts that are
 intrusive and unwanted. Such **obsessions** include
unwanted **sexual** thoughts about family or children,
sexual orientation or appearing to be homosexual ,
or fears about engaging in **sexually** aggressive
behavior.
sexual obsessions with unwanted sexual thoughts,
often involving children,, family members,
animals, violence, or even religious figures. These
sexual obsessions may involve same sex activities
or fear of changing sexual orientation.
 It is important to recognize that people with sexual

obsessions find their thoughts immoral and do not wish to act them out and these thoughts are different from fantasies. The obsessions are unpleasant and provoke guilt, but the fantasies are enjoyable thoughts. As a result, these unpleasant thoughts cause distress   with unwanted emotions, such as lust, disgust, anger, and frequently guilt. These obsessions can lead to depression, difficulties concentrating, and anxiety. The sexual obsessions are abnormal sexual thoughts and people suffering from these unwanted thoughts should keep their mind occupied by healthy activities and seek professional help .

40) Sexual addiction

The people with sexual addiction are obsessed with sex and have an intense sexual drive. They want to have sexual activities all the time. A person with **Sex addiction** can be a highly dangerous and destructive condition. Like any other addition , **drug** or **alcohol dependence**, it affects the addict's mental health, personal relationships, quality of life, and safety. It is common, but is often not diagnosed. Their thoughts are dominated by sexual activity, to the point where this affects other activities and interactions. If these urges become uncontrollable, the person can have difficulty functioning in social situations.

People with sexual addiction can be either male or female and

their lives are consumed with the sexual thoughts and sexual activity. The sooner they seek professional help for their addiction the better the chances are for getting rid of their addiction.

41)PROSTITUTION, in other words PAYING FOR SEX

Prostitution is the business or practice of engaging in sexual activity in exchange for payment. Prostitution is sometimes described as sexual services, commercial sex or, hooking and the women practicing it are called hookers. It is also known as "the world's oldest profession ". Prostitution has been practiced since the antiquity and is mention in the bible and other ancient books.
Several countries have laws against prostitution but that does not prevent the prostitutes and organized crime to practice their profession. In other progressive countries have legalized prostitution with regular health checks of the people practicing

it , in order to prevent the spread of sexual transmitted diseases and collect taxes from them. Most of the sex trade workers, are females but there   male prostitutes as well. Some of them are driven to the sex trade voluntary but most of them are the victims of sexual abuse and organized crime. **Prostitution** is defined as a criminal act that includes the sex trade, barter, or exchange of sexual acts with the hopes of the receipt of economic gain or opportunity. The sexual acts expressed within legislation addressing the act of **Prostitution** can include copulation, stimulation,   intercourse or other sexual acts.

Prostitution in any community strongly affect those communities

in a bad way , by contributing to the objectification of women and using the prostitutes as mere sex objects. It also increases the criminal activities and the violence against women.

The most negative effects of prostitution are: sexual transmitted and other venereal diseases, high risk of unwanted pregnancies, high risk of injuries from violent and dangerous clients, risk of alcohol and drug addictions , guild and depression and an increase in violent sexual crimes and abuse. Unfortunately many women and children involved in prostitution are the victims of sexual

abuse and sexual trafficking.
There are no social benefits of prostitution and it should
Be legalized to protect women and other sex trade workers
from   abuse and violence. It will also reduce or lessen the spread of sexually transmitted diseases, plus it can generate Taxes for the government from their businesses .
If there was no demand it would not be any prostitution, but it seems that there is great demand of prostitution in all the countries regardless if it is legal or illegal.
Prostitution is an abnormal sexual act no matter if they use the male penis and female vagina for their sexual activity.
 Considering the many risks involved in using the services of prostitutes one can wonder why take such risk for a passing pleasure and paying good money for it. But then again people make their choices and their health and their wallet pay the price..

42) SEXUAL ABUSE

Sexual abuse is an unwanted sexual activity, with perpetrators using force, making threats or taking advantage of victims not able to give consent. Sometimes the victims and the perpetrators know each other. Sexual abuse, also referred to as molestation, is abusive sexual behavior by one person upon another. It is often perpetrated using force or by taking advantage of another. When force is immediate, of short duration, or infrequent, it is called sexual assault. The offender is referred to as a sexual abuser or molester.
While a sexual abuser can be anyone, many sexual

abusers share **certain traits**. Child abuse offenders have **personality characteristics** that facilitate the sexual abuse of children. For example, child abusers are attracted to children sexually and are willing to act on these impulses.
Immediate reactions to sexual abuse include shock, fear terror or disbelief. Long-term symptoms include anxiety, fear or post-traumatic stress disorder.
Sexual abuse can happen to anyone but mostly occur in young children and disadvantaged people. The abuse can occur anywhere

that the abuser has access to the abused. It can happen once or can be chronic sexual abuse. And the people affected by sexual abuse can have life long   suffering .
Sexual abuse is a growing phenomenon and many times goes unreported for years. In the last few years many people came out and reported these unwanted sexual abuses   starting the "ME TOO MOVEMENT".   Many famous and rich people were named as sexual abusers and perpetrator .
Anyone that was a victim of sexual abuse, should report it to the authorities even if it is many years later. That is the only way to stop the sexual predators. Name them, shame them prosecute them and register them in the national registry of

sexual predators.

It is obvious that the sexual abuse can never be considered as a normal sexual act, even if the sexual activity is male penis to female vagina. The sexual abuse of anybody is an abnormal sexual activity and a criminal act.

There was a story on the television of a man who abducted three young women and he kept them chained in his home basement for a few years. During that time of their captivity he was sexually abusing them and one of the girls got pregnant and she had a baby. Eventually one of the girls escaped and she called the police and that deviant man was arrested . He eventually committed suicide while in custody, before even going to trial. There are many other cases of sexual abuse in the news papers and televisions. It seems that humans commit heinous sexual criminal acts , something that the other animals of the animal kingdom never do.

<u>Perhaps humans have a lot to learn from the other animals about normal sexual behavior. The animals never abuse sexually other animals.</u>

If you are the victim of any abuse, sexually or otherwise, just remember this, it was not your fault. You were the victim of that abuse and the sooner you report that abuse the sooner you will get help and free yourself from any unintentional

guilt. Do the right thing that   so many other
abused people are doing with the "ME TOO
MOVEMENT".

43) SEX Trafficking

Sex trafficking is a criminal activity that involves
mainly young girls abused and exploited by
criminals   for sexual prostitution.
Human sex trafficking is the most common form of
modern slavery and   the number of domestic and
international victims are in the millions, mostly
females and children enslaved in the commercial
sex industry for little or no money. They usually
illegally transport people from one country to
another for the purpose of sexual exploitation.
Sex trafficking is often under-reported, under-
estimated and largely misunderstood.   Sex
trafficking occurs when exploiting someone
through force, fraud or coercion for another
person's financial gain. Sex traffickers move their
vulnerable victims from country to country and
from city to city as their slaves, for the purpose of
forcing them to commit sexual acts for the
economic gain of their traffickers. Sex traffickers

even buy and sell their victims like any other
commodity.
Traffickers are using the Internet and other social
means as a way to target unsuspecting and
vulnerable youth for their own personal financial
gain..
Sex trafficking is a criminal activity taking
advantage of vulnerable people and it is one of
fastest growing crimes all over the world.
All the sexual activities derived from the illegal
sex trafficking are abnormal sexual acts . These
criminal activities should be reported to the local
and international authorities for the punishment of
the criminals and free the   sexually abused people.
If you are the victim of sex trafficking , no matter
if you are legally or illegally in the country you
were transported, report your masters, the sex
traffickers , to the local authorities so that you and
society get rid of these scum's control. The
authorities usually provide, legal, moral and
financial support for the victims of   such an abuse.

44) SEXUAL SLAVERY

One might think, that this is the twenty first century
and that there are no more slave people on planet
earth. But that is not the case, slavery of people is
still alive and thriving in all parts of the world.

People are bought and sold by others like any other commodity. People are forced into slavery sometimes by poor choices , economic circumstances, coerced ,or forceful entrapment . Sexual slavery and sexual exploitation is attaching the right of ownership over one or more persons with the intent of coercing or otherwise forcing them to engage in sexual activities. This includes forced labor, reducing a person to a servile status and sex trafficking persons, such as the sexual trafficking of children and women. The slaves and their masters might have a good relationship for mutual economic benefit , or it might be just forced slavery where women, children and even grown up men are forced into   sexual slavery for the sole benefit of their masters.

Whatever the situation is and no matter what type of sexual acts they perform, this is unacceptable and abnormal sexual acts , even if it is vagina-penis sexual acts. These sexual acts are abnormal and deplorable. These acts have nothing to do with natural normal sexual act for procreation. These sexual acts is the abuse of human beings both mentally and physically for the economic benefit of their masters. These acts are not only abnormal sexual acts but illegal as well and the governments of all countries should take the necessary measures to end this deplorable situation and punish severely the so called masters by sending them to prisons for long time.

If you are the victim of slavery, report your masters
to the local authorities so that you and society get
rid of these scum's control. Remember that it was
not your fault. You were the victim of that situation
and the sooner you report that to the authorities the
sooner you will get help.

45) SEXUAL ABUSE AND MENTAL ILLNESS

Since the sexual revolution in the 1960's and
1970's the sexual abuse has dramatically increase.
The sexual **revolution** also known as a time of
"sexual liberation" was a social movement that
challenged traditional codes of behavior related to
sexuality and interpersonal relationships. There was
always some sexual abuse but by dismantling the
traditional codes of behavior related to sexuality,
an open season of sexual abuse began , especially
against the young and the vulnerable.
The sexual abuse is usually associated with mental
and physical abuse and has detrimental effects on
the lives of the abused victims.
As a result of the sexual abuses there are long term

effects on those sexually abused. The most obvious effect is **psychological harm** which includes, **depression, post traumatic stress disorder, behavioral problems**, including **sexualized behavior, poor self-esteem, academic problems and suicide**. Every year more and more people are having mental problems from sexual , mental and physical abuse. Many lives are destroyed by these abuses.

The society has to do something about this disturbing trend. The abuses are criminal acts and society should have laws to punish severely those that abuse others. The society's courts   should send a message that the society will not tolerate the sexual, physical and mental abuse of its citizens by anyone , no matter what

position they have in society.

The parents and the school system should teach kids from a young age to treat each other with respect and report any abuse to the proper authorities. They should bring back civility and "the golden rule" in the school teachings.

Finally if you are the victim of such an assault, no matter how many years ago it happened , speak out and report that abuse, or even sue for damages the perpetrator for that abuse. That is the only way to stop that perpetrator from harming other people,

plus to empower you not to feel a victim anymore.
I am glad that the "me too" movement was born
to put an end to any abuse no matter how long ago
it happened .
Sexual abuse can happen to any one even by their
own father or other relatives.
Here is an excerpt from a sexual abuse story
published in the internet about a father sexually
abusing his daughters!!!!!!

""Stuff of nightmares': Crown wants 29 years for
father who sexually abused daughters at rural
compound
"RCMP arrested the man in late 2016 after a tip
from an extended family member. Court heard the
man offered his teenaged daughter up for sex with
strangers on the internet — filming, directing and
even participating in one of the rapes. He later
forced the daughter to watch video of the
assaults.+" September 17,2019
The prosecutor was asking the court for   a
sentencing of big jail time and emphasized that
by saying, "I understand I am asking for an
unprecedented sentence," she told Court , "But
with respect, sir, this man is an unprecedented
offender."
Karla told Ouellette the sentence he passes "must
tell this offender and anyone like him that this type
of carnage will not be tolerated. This is the stuff of

nightmares. The difference is for the complainants and the family — they don't get to wake up."

During a video of one of the incidents, the accused "served (his daughter) up to strangers," Karla said, adding he could be heard telling the men they could be "aggressive" as long as they did not leave permanent marks or pull out her hair. She noted that despite being tied up, "she doesn't scream. Can you imagine what must have been done to this human soul that …. she does not make a sound?"
"""

Reading stories like this makes you wonder what type of a human person he is , if you can call him human, that can do such a heinous crime against his own daughters? And one may wonder , if there is any safe place for kids to be kids anymore?
If you were the victim of such an abuse report it to the authorities as soon as possible to get the help you need and deserve.

46) THE HUGE SEXUAL INDUSTRY

The sexual industry is a huge industry worth billions of dollars. The sex industry consists of businesses that either directly or indirectly provide sex-related products and services and adult entertainment. The industry includes activities involving direct provision of sexual services, such as prostitution, strip clubs, host and hostess clubs and sex-related pastimes, such as pornography, sex-oriented men's magazines, sex movies, sex toys and fetish and bondage and submission. Many sex workers are forced or coerced into the sex industry.

The main forms of the sex industry are street prostitution, escort services, child prostitution, internet chat rooms, male prostitution, sex tourism and more.

 Despite the advancement of human civilization and human rights, the problem of human slavery and sexual abuse continues to grow and is rampant in all the countries.

The sex industry is controlled by the underworld in most major cities. In some major cities you can see everywhere signs for

sex services. Female sex workers walking in the street corners, bright signs for massage parlors , night clubs and other establishments. Most of the sex workers are lured or force into the trade. Many sex workers are the victims of sex trafficking and sex slavery. The governments efforts to put an end to the sex trafficking and sex slavery is not effective.

It is obvious that sexual activities of the sex industry is an abnormal sexual activity for economic gains of the people running the sex industry.

47) History of the sex trade
The history of the sex trade is as old as humanity. The sex trade can be traced back to antiquity, the Sumerians and Babylonians. It flourished in the big cities during the middle ages in most parts of the world. It was considered sinful by all religious entities which they were promoting the family values. Regulations against the sex trade increased across Europe after the outbreak of syphilis in Naples during the fifteenth century. Sex trafficking increased across the world during the 19th century. The sex trade increased tremendously in the latter half of the 20th century as a result of globalization and western tourism.
Unfortunately the sex trade is here to stay and the governments should take the necessary measures to protect the victims of the sex trade globally. The increase of the sex trade so is the transition of the sexually transmitted diseases.

48) OTHER PARAPHILIAS OF DEVIANT SEXUAL ACTIVITY

There are a lot of abnormal and deviant sexual

activities called paraphilias. We talked about some of them but still there all sorts of abnormal sexual preferences by humans, and most of them are illegal and immoral .

A paraphilia is a condition in which a person's sexual arousal and gratification depend on fantasizing about or engaging in sexual behavior that is atypical and extreme. A paraphilia is considered a disorder when it causes distress or threatens to harm themselves or someone else. Paraphilias include sexual behaviors society view as distasteful, unusual, or abnormal.. Some of the behaviors are illegal, and individuals with those disorders often have legal problems as well. Paraphilic Disorders may include sexual acts such as those involving dead people, urine, feces, enemas, or obscene phone calls, animals and other extreme abnormal sexual preferences.

It is obvious that many of these activities you can encounter them only in humans and never in other animals. Humans have a lot to learn about the normal sexual behavior of animals and their way of life in general.

49) SEXUAL EDUCATION IN SCHOOLS

Sex **education** should be **taught** in high **schools**, as well as in the earlier years of **education**. Sex **education** can **teach** people of all

ages the consequences and responsibilities of engaging in **sexual** activities. Sex **education** should be **taught** in every **public** and private school .

The schools should teach the students that the only normal sexual activity is the male penis to female vagina and that the normal sexual activity is the nature's way for procreation. They should also teach them not to rush into any sexual activity before their bodies is mature enough and are both mentally and physically to face any consequences of their actions. Sex is not about fun and pleasure, it has it's responsibilities and consequences. It is normal not to have sex before you are ready to face the responsibilities of the any sexual activity. The schools should teach the kids the truth about the dangers associated with any sexual activity.

Studies show that sex education is **most effective** when it is implemented **prior to the onset of sexual activity**, and when it combines both abstinence and contraceptive information.
 Sex education will empower the students to make informed decisions about sex and sex dangers. Studies have not found that sex education encourages sexual experimentation or increased involvement in sexual activity.
Sex education should encourage abstinence until their bodies are sexually mature and even then not to rush into anything that are not prepared to face the consequences like pregnancy and sexually transmitted diseases.

School sex education should teach the kids the truth about sex , vagina sex, anal sex , and any other type of sex and never ever bend the truth to satisfy any new FAD or the few that are always loud and demand that their way of life is right. They should teach the kids about the role the males and females have in the procreation process. The gifts they have from nature as males the penis and females the vagina. They should emphasize that any sexual act has its consequences and that they should not rush into anything before they grow up and are mature enough to take care of their responsibilities. Sex is a serious matter with serious consequences. Any

sexual activity can be dangerous to their health from the sexual transmitted diseases.
They should teach them that if they want to be mothers or fathers someday ,that they have to be very careful about their sex life . With any sexual activity there is a risk   of serious infections which can cause serious diseases including cancer and sterility.

Sex is not always about fun and pleasure, sex is a serious business
  with serious consequences, like pregnancy to the females, and potential serious health risks to every one engaging in any sexual activity .

The school sex education should be done separate for boys and girls so that kids are not embarrassed to ask questions. Although the sex education is done separately for boys and girls, they should teach both boys and girls about the anatomy and physiology of both sexes.

50) Sex education at home

Sex education should start at home by the parents. It is the parents responsibility to teach their kids about sex and their life values.

The parents should teach their kids from an early age about their private parts with the normal names of each sexual organ. They should also teach them that their private sex organs are private and that nobody else should tough them there. If anybody tries to touch their privates parts , they should report it to their parents right away. Of course they should tell them that the kids should never touch the private parts of other kids or grown ups.

They should also teach their kids why boys and girls sexual organs are different and be proud of what they got, it is a priceless gift from nature. Nature provides the girls with their sex organs and the boys with their sex organs and when the grow up they will be able to have babies of their own. They should teach boys that their sexual organs, when they grow up and are mature enough

will produce the spermatozoa , In other words the seeds that when combined with the mature eggs of the women will produce their babies.

They should teach the girls that although nature did not give them a penis, nature gave them the greatest gift of all, the ability to make babies.

Teach them that their sexual organs are different than the boys but they have the ability to produce eggs and when the eggs combine with sperm of boys when they grow up they will procreate a new life, new babies.

They should also teach the kids that in order to be able to have their own kids someday, they should take good care of themselves and   not experiment with any sexual activity until they are mature   and ready to face the responsibilities of having babies. Parents should answer any questions that their kids might ask, with clarity and honesty.

The parents should warned their kids about the sexual predators and tell them to avoid talking to strangers and that even friends of the family should not engage with them in any physical contact involving their private parts.

<u>Parents should be on the look out for possible child molesters and predators among their friend, neighbors   and relatives.</u> Many kids are sexually abused by family friends, neighbors   and relatives.

.

<u>The parents responsibility is to protect their kids and not to worry if they will offend the deviant behavior of their friends or relatives.</u>

They should also warn them about the dangers of the internet and they should never chat with

strangers in chat rooms and never send any pictures of themselves nude or   with clothes because you never know where those pictures will end up…
They should also tell them about bullying and that they can come to them for help with any questions or concerns they might

have.
<u>Kids need to know that their parents are their to protect them from any danger or threat.</u>

Encourage them to ask any question they might have and tell them the truth if they ask   Where do the babies come from?
If they ask where do the babies come from, just tell them the truth; from their mothers womb and explain to them that women have the exclusive privilege to make babies and that the men have the privilege to produce the seeds that enable women to have babies.

<u>How are babies made? A seed from the daddy and an egg from the mommy join together to create a new baby in the mommy's tummy.</u>

That's how the baby is made and it grows in a special sack in the mother's womb until it is ready

to come out and start a new life.
The parents should always answer any question
their kids ask them. That is the only way to teach
your kids the values you want them to have.

51) SEXUAL EDUCATION FOR ALL

It is obvious that all people need to have sex
education. It does not mean that grown ups know
everything about sex and the risks involved. When
people do not know all the facts about the pros
and the cons of any sexual activity they cannot
make   an informed decision.
 Many adults commit heinous sexual crimes
against other people , including young children or
they are the victims or other adults. With the
advent of the internet, everybody can get
information about anything, and all they have to do
is just search the internet. The information is there
for everybody to read and increase his or her
knowledge about any subject including sex. By
getting all the information , you can make an
informed decision and especially to protect the
young and the vulnerable.

People can learn a lot about normal sexual behavior

by observing the animals' sexual behavior . The
animals have sex just for procreation and never
for recreation and that's what nature had in mind
when   it created the male and female sex organs in
all animals including humans.
People of all ages, even   educated people that they
are supposed to know that sex is for procreation ,
have been accused of abnormal sexual abuse of
others including children.
There is need to educate young and old about the
sex and that any sexual act should be a consensual
act and never used to use or sexually abuse
anybody, especially the most vulnerable members
of society, the children .

52) HOW TO PROTECT KIDS FROM SEXUAL PREDATORS

There are sexual predators everywhere ready to
lure kids for their abnormal sexual acts and it is
up to parents and society to empower the kids
with the necessary knowledge to avoid any sexual
abuse.
The parents should teach their kids from an early
age about their private parts with the normal
names of each sexual organ. They should also
teach them that their private sex organs are private
and that nobody else should tough them there. If

anybody tries to touch their privates, they should report it to their parents right away. Of course they should tell them that the kids should never touch the private parts of other kids or grown ups.
As soon as children start talking, to tell them that , 'your body is yours alone, and no one should touch your body, and they should not touch anybody's else body if they ask them to so. Children are taught to be polite and say "yes, please" and "thank you"; but they should also be taught to say "no" when they don't want to be affectionate, or do anything they do not want to do..
They should talk not to strangers and definitely they should never embrace or hug any strangers and even people they know if they do not want to.
They should also

tell them to report to the parents if any family friend or relative try to touch them inappropriately .

<u>Parents should be on the look out for possible child molesters and predators among their friend, neighbors and relatives</u>. Many kids are sexually abused by family friends, neighbors   and relatives. The parents responsibility is to protect their kids and not to worry if they will offend the deviant behavior of their friends or relatives.

They should also warn them about the dangers of
the internet and they should never chat with
strangers in chat rooms and never send any
pictures of themselves nude or   with clothes
because you never know where those pictures will
end up…

53) HOW TO PROTECT THE VULNERABLE FROM SEXUAL AND PHYSICAL ABUSE

Many vulnerable people are abused daily by the
people that they were hired to look after them.
Kids under the care of care givers, people with
mental of physical disabilities and other vulnerable
people are abused , mentally, physically or
emotionally. Some of these abuses are going
unrecognized and unreported .
It is up to the people that love and   care about their
loved ones to try to prevent, recognize and report
such abuses. There were reports in the media that
the relatives of some vulnerable people were able
to   recognize and report the abusers by installing
cameras In the room of their loved ones. I think
this is the best way to catch the abusers of the
vulnerable people. When you have the proof
report it to authorities and fire the abuser
immediately.

54) HUMAN SEXUAL ACTIVITY VERSUS ANIMAL SEXUAL ACTIVITY:

who is right and who is wrong about sex? Humans' sexual activities or animals sexual activity? You might be surprised …

In a way the animals are lucky that they do not have any hang ups about sexual activities. The animals follow instinctively the nature's way about the normal sexual activity. They know when it is time to have sex and the reason why they engage in sexual activity.: to produce the next generation of their kind. The animals have sex only when the female animal is mature and ready to have babies, and only when the female is in heat, in other words she is ready to have sex and conceive. If the female animal is not ready to conceive, she will not have sex with any male animal , period. In reality the sex life of the animals is perfect and that is the ideal normal sexual activity , something that the humans have a lot to learn from.

Humans on the other hand have confused ideas about sex, they even forgot what the sexual activity is for. Humans think the sexual activity is a sport of some sort and try to have as much sex as possible and at any time. Humans do not have sex just for procreation but mostly for recreation. They do not care if the female is mature enough or she is in heat and ready to conceive.

Humans have sexual activities not only with their sexual organs but they use non sexual parts of their bodies and even foreign objects for their sexual activities and pleasures. It is an open season for sexual activities at anytime , anywhere at any place and with no regard to health and safety. Many serious diseases are transmitted from person to person with normal and abnormal

sexual activities with detrimental effects on those affected. Humans even use sexual activities for economic gain for them or others . They created huge sex industries for making money and have nothing to do with the actual normal purpose of sex, procreation.

In short humans lost their ways and they are confused about sex and sexual acts . Humans forgot what is the real purpose of sex, which is for procreation and it was never intended for recreation.

Humans have a lot to learn about sex from studying the animals sexual activities and

**behavior.**
**And if human follow the animal's example about**
**sex , the world will be a better place with less**
**violence and criminal activities.**

55) CONCLUSION

In conclusion there is only one normal sexual act, the male penis to female vagina intercourse. The normal sexual activity is for procreation and it was never intended for recreation. However , the male penis to female vagina sexual intercourse is always a normal sexual activity ,, no matter if it is just for procreation or sexual pleasure ,provided it is consensual by both parties. Besides not every normal sexual activity yields a baby.

Nature with all its wisdom decides when a baby will be produced and humans while keep trying to produce babies they are hooked on the   sexual pleasure so much, so that they even forgot the real purpose of the sexual act. Humans in their quest to have as much sexual pleasure as possible started using their sexual organs with other parts of the body or even created an industry of sexual toys. That's how the abnormal sexual acts and the sex toys were invented for just sexual pleasure. That is why these sexual acts are abnormal sexual activities, they are just for pleasure and not for what the nature had in mind , the procreation. Besides these abnormal sexual acts can cause infections and other diseases that can cause the normal sexual organs to become obsolete and incapable of performing their intended function, the creation of babies. Many people are either ignorant of the risks of the abnormal sexual activities or they are just interesting to have as much sexual pleasure as possible and they ignore the potential health risks. By the time they realize the enormous health damage that those abnormal activities are doing to their sexual organs and their health, it is too late.

56) EPILOGUE

In the animal world there are no sexual hang-ups about their sexual activity. Their sexual activities is just for procreation and nothing else. As a result of their normal sexual activities they do not suffer from any sexual insecurities, abnormal sexual ambiguities or the maladies that human are affected.

Humans on the other hand they forgot the real purpose of the sexual activity , they are confused and have a lot of hang-ups about their sexual activities. Humans sexually abuse others including the young and vulnerable something that other animals never do. As a result of that, they are suffering the consequences, Sexual transmitted diseases, mental and physical diseases and other

infections   that ravage their health and sexual
organs dysfunction including sterility.. They
created multibillion dollars sex industries just
for recreation at the peril of procreation. Humans
are heading the wrong direction with their sexual
activities and they can learn a lot from the sexual
activities of the other animals, before it is too late
for the human race.

Humans have to realize that there is only one
normal sexual activity, the man penis to the female
vagina, whether is done for procreation or
pleasure. Any other sexual activity, according to
the abnormal psychology, is an abnormal and
deviant sexual activity, called paraphilias . Any
one having any doubts , they can look it up for
themselves.

Consenting adults can do whatever they want in the
privacy of their bedrooms as long as they do not
use or sexually abuse others without their consent.
When their health pay the price for their abnormal
sexual activities , they will have nobody else to
blame but themselves.

57) THE SEEDS OF LIFE

Something to think about the seeds of life, plant seeds, frog seeds and human seeds, the spermatozoa

Similarities of the life of the spermatozoa and the frog's tadpole in their journey to become a human baby from the spermatozoa and a frog from the tadpole, and of course the plants seeds to plants..

Long before they started using ddt and other chemicals to control mosquitoes and other pests in the creeks and standing waters, there were a lot of frogs laying their eggs in those waters. You could see a jelly like sack full of frog eggs attached at the shallow area of the waters. In a few weeks the eggs were hatching and the tadpoles were emerging from the frog's eggs. The tadpoles look exactly like the human spermatozoa as seen under the microscope. The tadpoles were moving around collecting their nutritional food from the waters and exercising. With time a metamorphosis was taking place with tadpoles gradually developing the frog's head and growing their four legs. Eventually the tadpoles were transformed into frogs and their tail was shed off as they did not need it to swim any more .

The tadpole and the human spermatozoa look exactly the same and they go through the same transformation in their quest to become the final animal, the frog for the tadpole and the human baby for the sperm. The tadpole uses the creek waters to feed and develop but the sperm has more nutritional needs so it has to be attached on the uterine wall to get all the nutritional needs from the mother .

The sperm enters the female egg which has the nutrition for his survival and growth. The human egg acts as the waters of the

creek where the tadpole spends his transformation period. The sperm needs a lot of nutrition for growth and transformation and since the human egg does not have all the nutritional needs for the sperm the egg attaches itself to the uterine wall to get all the nutritional needs of the developing baby from the mother. The egg that contains the sperm fills up with the amniotic fluid where the

growing baby will swim and keep growing until
the new baby develops his head arms and legs and
it is ready to come as a new human being. Both
the tadpole and the spermatozoa start with the
same shape and through the metamorphosis they
transform into a frog from the tadpole and to a
human baby from the spermatozoa. The tadpole
uses the water of the lagoon as his growing
environment and the spermatozoa uses the
amniotic fluid for his growing environment for his
metamorphosis. The tadpole needs only a few
weeks for his metamorphosis and the spermatozoa
needs nine months of his metamorphosis and his
transformation into a human baby.

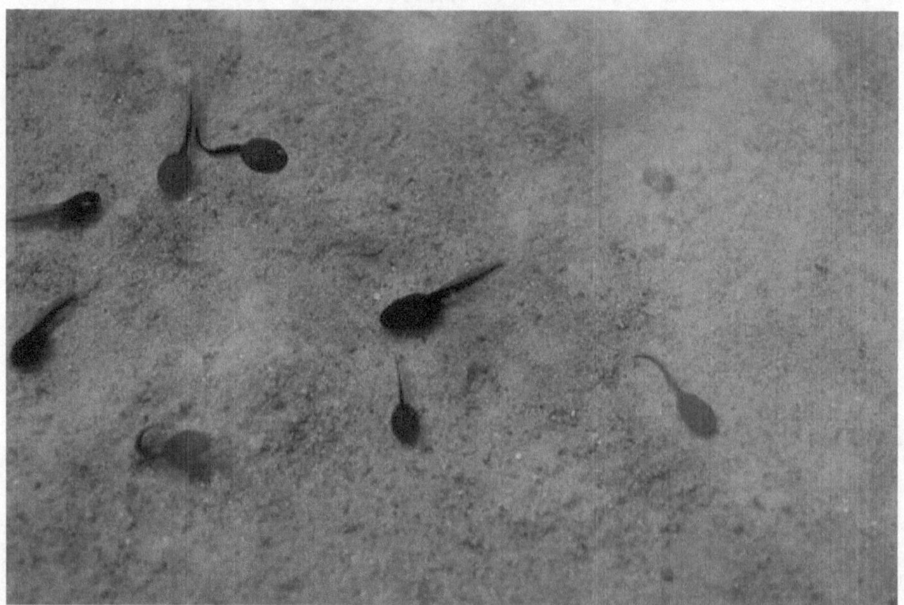

Tadpoles in water

tadpoles 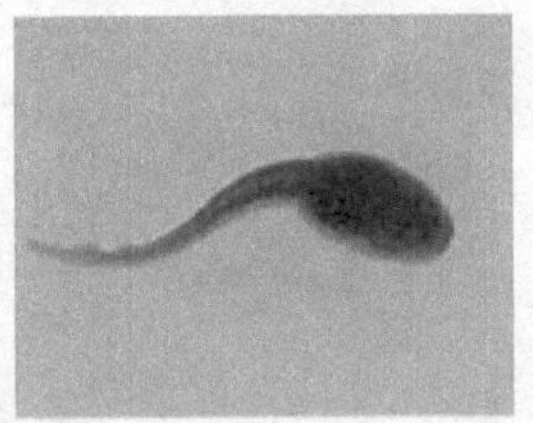

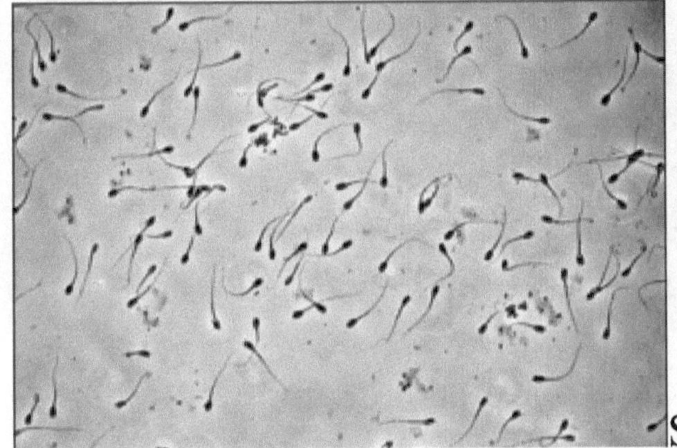
Spermatozoa as seen under the microscope. Look how similar to tadpoles look.

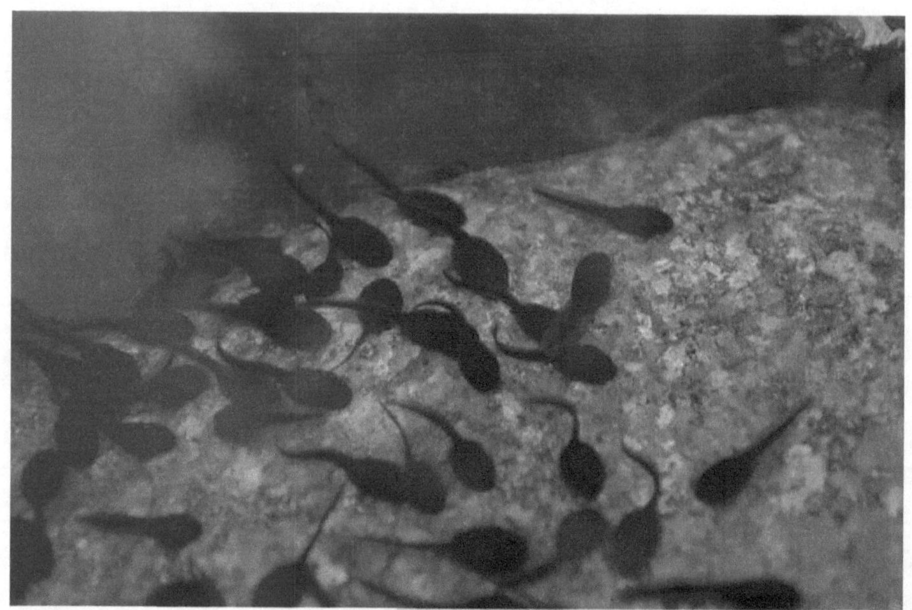

tadpoles   in a lagoon after they hatched

Both tadpoles and the spermatozoa go though the same

metamorphosis and transformation to reach their
final destination as a fully developed frog from the
tadpole and a fully developed human baby from
the spermatozoa. Understand their similarities and
transformation and you understand how nature
works for all living creatures.

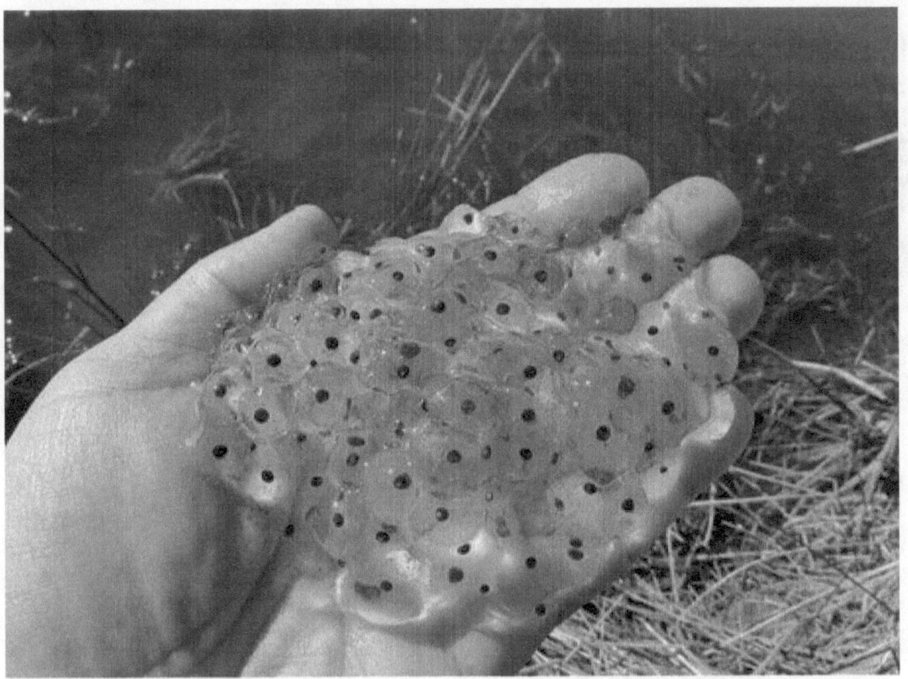

Frog's eggs in a jelly like sack before they hatch and emerge as tadpoles.

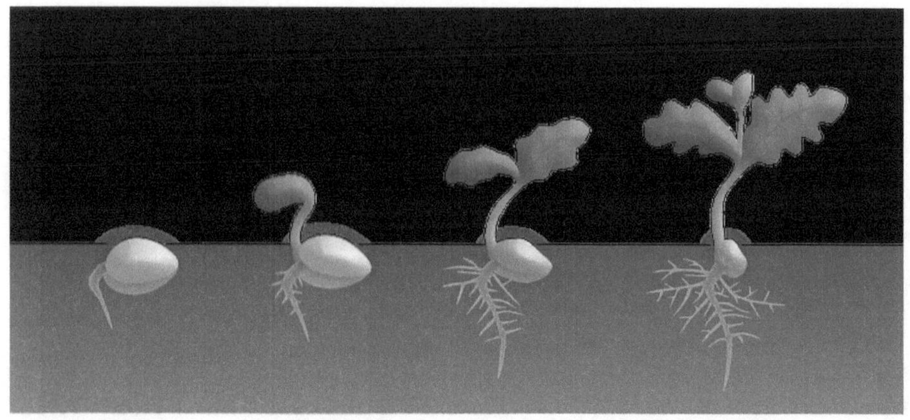

Plant seeds germinating and transforming into a tree.

 Look how this germinating seed looks like a

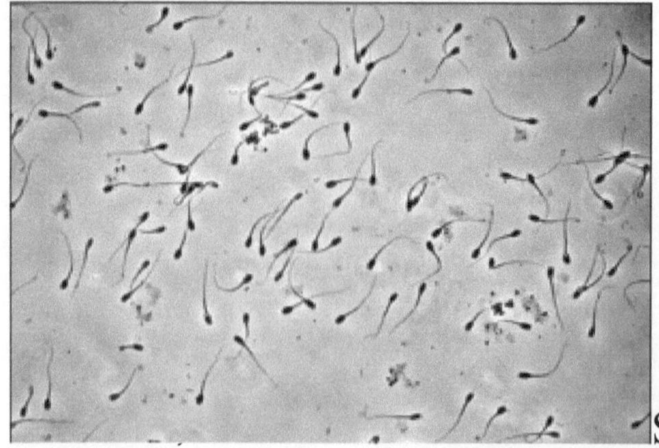

tadpole As seen swimming in water, Which will transform into a frog

Spermatozoa the human seeds, as seen under the microscope, They will transform into human babies.

The plants' seeds ,the tadpoles and the
spermatozoa go though the same metamorphosis
and transformation to reach their final
transformation, as a tree from the tree seed, as a
fully developed frog from the tadpole and a fully
developed human baby from the spermatozoa.
All the seeds , spermatozoa in humans, seeds in
plants, tadpoles of frogs, have everything
necessary to develop and transform into a baby
from the spermatozoa, seeds into a plant, tadpoles
into frogs provided they find a fertile ground. The
human spermatozoa need fertile ground in the
female egg, the plant seeds need fertile soil and
the tadpoles need standing water with lots of
nutrients in it .
Understand their similarities and transformation
and you understand how nature works for all
living creatures.

Book description.

This book is like a sex manual for normal and

abnormal sexual activities.
This book delves into the normal sexual activities of humans
This book is about the abnormal sexual activities of humans.
In this book you will read everything about sex both normal and abnormal and deviant.
In this book you will read the story of the " pregnant man".
In this book you will read about sexual abuses and what do about it. In this book you will read   about sex education at home and at school. In this book you will read about the sexual habits of animals and how humans can learn from the normal sexual activity of animals. This book is for everyone that has questions about normal and abnormal sexual activities .
Sex: the good , the bad and the ugly. It is all explained in simple language.
Normal sexual activities will give you pleasure and kids.
Abnormal sexual activities will cause mental and physical grief.
In this book you will read about the similarities that all live seeds have, the spermatozoa, the tadpole and the plants seeds.
 Read this book just out of curiosity to learn about the normal and abnormal sexual activities. It might help you to avoid some risky and dangerous to

your health sexual activities.

From the inside cover:
After finishing reading this book, give to someone
else to expand their knowledge about normal and
abnormal sexual activities. It might help them
make informed decisions and avoid risky sexual
activities that might cause harm to their health.
Knowledge is to be shared for the benefit all.

From the author.
Nature with all its wisdom provided all animals
with the necessary tools, their sex organs, for
procreation and the renewal of their kind. All
animals, in the animal kingdom, except humans,
follow the natures rules and practice only the
normal sexual activities for the sole purpose of
procreation . Some   Humans on the other hand
forgot the true purpose of sex and started using all
sorts of abnormal sexual activities with severe
health consequences, including sterility . As time
goes by more and more humans are attracted to
these abnormal sexual activities at the detriment of
their health and even the survival of the human
race.
There is only one normal sexual activity both for
procreation and sexual pleasure, the male penis to
the female vagina. Any other sexual activity is an
abnormal sexual activity with severe health
consequences including sterility and it puts at risk
the whole   survival of the human race.
Whatever consenting adults do in the privacy of
their homes is their business and nobody's else.
Ultimately people are free to make their own

choices and responsible for their actions. If their health pay the price for those choices, at least hey have no one else to blame for the consequences .

There is a need for sexual education of all people, including the young and the old, and this is the purpose of this book. To educate and empower people about normal and abnormal sexual activities, to make informed decisions and avoid the perils of risky sexual activities if they so choose to do.
Ultimately people make their own choices and they are responsible for the consequences of those decisions.